WHEN YOUR

PAIN

FLARES UP

*Easy, Proven Techniques
for Managing Chronic Pain*

PAIN MANAGEMENT CENTER, FAIRVIEW HEALTH SERVICES

Fairview Press · Minneapolis

Fairview Press is a division of Fairview Health Services, a community-focused health system providing a complete range of services, from the prevention of illness and injury to care for the most complex medical conditions.

Library of Congress Cataloging-in-Publication Data
When your pain flares up : easy, proven techniques for managing chronic pain / Pain Management Center, Fairview Health Services.
    p. cm.
Includes bibliographical references.
 ISBN 1-57749-120-3 (trade paperback : alk. paper)
1. Chronic pain--Popular works. I. Fairview Health Services. Pain Management Center.
RB127 .W475 2002
616'.0472--dc21

                            2002151086

First printing: December 2002
Printed in the United States of America
05 04 03 02   6 5 4 3 2 1

Interior by Dorie McClelland, Spring Book Design
Edited by Barbara St. Marie, MA, ANP, GNP; Susan Arnold, BA, RN, CHTP
Cover image: Digital Imagery © copyright 2001 PhotoDisc, Inc.
Funding and support for this book provided by Fairview Auxiliary.

Disclaimer

For a free current catalog of Fairview Press titles, please call toll-free 1-800-544-8207. Or visit our Web site at www.fairviewpress.org.

Contents

Introduction

Pain flare (a temporary escalation in pain) is poorly understood, yet all too familiar to people with chronic pain. A pain flare may have various causes, including physical activity, body positioning, weather pattern changes, stress, sleep disruption, and viruses, to name a few.

Those who have chronic pain often participate in a complex regimen of medications, stimulators, chiropractic adjustments, physical therapy stretches, and exercises. Even when they do all the right things, however, a pain flare may still occur.

A flare is similar in location and quality to your usual chronic pain. The difference is the severity. When pain is more severe, fear is the natural response, which leads to worry, stress, and more pain.

This book is intended to help individuals achieve pain relief during a pain flare. In the pages that follow, you will find a number of helpful pain management techniques. Everyone responds differently to these techniques, so you may want to try several methods or use a combination. By learning to control your view of and reaction to pain, you will take an important step in achieving pain relief. At the same time, taking an active role in working with the pain will help you control your response to it.

While prescription pain relievers can be helpful, they are not to be relied on exclusively. An overreliance on pain medication may become problematic, especially if you believe that medication is the only thing that works. For this reason, it's essential to develop a method of pain management—one that does not rely solely on medication.

In our experience, when individuals make these pain management techniques a part of their daily schedule, they see an improvement in their condition. Learning and practicing these techniques can be labor intensive, but the rewards are well worth the time and effort. In other words, how well you do depends on the effort you're willing to invest in yourself.

We believe that the self-care tools described in this book will empower you. Read this book all the way through, then ask yourself: If I have a pain flare, what will I do? Prepare yourself for a pain flare by writing out a plan. You will find a pain flare worksheet at the back of this book.

Relaxation and the Power of the Mind

Many people consider relaxation to mean watching TV, napping, or hanging out. Therapeutic relaxation, however, means taking time out for yourself to clear away stress, preoccupation, and tension by focusing your awareness on this moment rather than on the past or future. The "relaxation response" can be accomplished not by demanding relaxation, but by learning to let go of stressful thoughts or by thinking pleasant thoughts.

The National Institutes of Health looked at a number of mental awareness techniques used in pain management. It found that "the evidence is strong for the effectiveness of these techniques in reducing chronic pain in a variety of medical conditions." Relaxation and other awareness techniques help with both short- and long-term pain management.

Most people are able to use their mind to alleviate, and sometimes prevent, a pain flare. Awareness techniques may not get rid of pain permanently, but they do give you more control over your pain. And, they do not require medication. Daily use of meditation and relaxation techniques can lead to progressively less pain over time, especially if used in conjunction with stretching, exercise, and stress management.

At first, learning to relax or meditate may feel uncomfortable to people who live busy, hectic lives. Many people feel they need to be doing something constantly, or they do not believe that they can relax and slow their busy minds. However, if you practice every day, you will learn to let go of the thoughts and emotions that continually pass through your mind. Letting go means giving your mind some time and space of its own without criticisms, judgments, or expectations. You can always get back to these things later.

Self-Comfort

In order to relax, you must first make yourself comfortable. Sit or lie down with a pillow, and experiment with different positions. Try placing the pillow under the knees, between the knees, or between the arms. Or, sit with pillow support either over your abdomen or behind your back, keeping your neck straight and arms well supported. If you get sore after being in one position, get up and walk around for a while.

Become a nonjudgmental observer of what is happening inside your body. Be just slightly aware of what is going on during relaxation or meditation; do not focus on goals you need to accomplish. By adopting a detached, watchful attitude, you give your body a chance to unwind. You are not telling your body that it has to "do something"; rather, you are simply allowing it to "be." As you begin to let go of expectations and judgments about what you are supposed to experience, you will find that you are able to relax.

No matter which awareness technique you use, you will eventually encounter the situation where your mind wanders off. You may begin to think about various problems that are coming up, or about events that happened in the past. The moment you start thinking about these things, you are no longer in the present. To continue relaxation, return your awareness to your breathing and let go of the thoughts or images that led you off course. Then, focus your awareness on the technique you are using. Really notice how your body feels as it relaxes. Focusing on the changes in your body will help you to stay in the present, which is a skill you can use anytime you want to reduce anxiety and stress.

Simply focus on what's happening right now, instead of projecting needlessly into the future or getting stuck in the past.

Awareness techniques include muscle relaxation exercises, autogenics training, breathing exercises, music relaxation, and visual imagery. Try them all to see which you like best. If you practice every day, you may find yourself feeling refreshed and able to engage in your activities with more energy, efficiency, and creativity.

Muscle Relaxation

These exercises will help you recognize the feeling of muscle tightness so you can appreciate the contrast between muscular tension and muscular relaxation. Perform these exercises in a quiet and comfortably warm room. Your movements should be slow and smooth, and you should breathe naturally throughout all the exercises.

Shoulder Shrugging

Sit in a chair and let your arms hang loosely at your sides. Shrug your shoulders and tighten the muscles as much as possible. Hold the position until the muscles of your neck and shoulders feel tight. Hold for a count of 5. Release the tension and let the shoulders drop. Repeat three times.

Head Circles

Sit in a chair and let your arms hang loosely. Allow your shoulders to relax and droop. Roll your head slowly to the side, then in a circle. Repeat three times in each direction.

Shoulder Rolls

Sitting in a chair with your arms resting at your sides, slowly roll one shoulder up and back, circling in one direction, then the other. Repeat three times for each shoulder, then do both shoulders together three times in each direction.

Arm and Fist Tightening

Lie on your back or sit in a chair, allowing your arms to rest at your sides. Clench your right fist tightly and bend the elbow. Hold for a count of 5. Release your fist and allow your arm to straighten slowly. Repeat three times with each arm.

Chest Tightening with Arms Overhead

Lie on your back with your arms spread out at your sides. Keeping your arms straight, slowly raise them above your chest, moving your palms toward one another until your hands meet. Press your palms together until you feel your chest muscles contract.

Hold for a count of 5. Gradually release the pressure and return your arms to your sides. Repeat three times.

General Muscle Relaxation

Have someone with a soothing voice read the directions into a tape recorder. This way you can close your eyes, get comfortable, and concentrate on the directions.

Exercise One

1. Let all your muscles go loose and heavy. Just settle back quietly and comfortably. Wrinkle up your forehead . . . then smooth it out. Picture the entire forehead and scalp becoming smoother and softer as you begin to relax. Now, frown and crease your brows and notice the tightness. . . . Let go of the tension again, softening the muscles. Tighten and then smooth out the forehead once more. Extend the softening into the temples and scalp. Close your eyes, gently, comfortably, and notice the relaxation.

2. Now, clench your jaws and teeth together. Study the tension throughout the jaws . . . then begin to relax your jaws. Let your lips part slightly. Appreciate the relaxation by breathing into it, allowing your jaws to soften.

3. Press your tongue hard against the roof of your mouth. Notice the tension. . . . Now press your lips together tighter and tighter. . . . Relax the lips, allowing your tongue, lips, roof of the mouth, and jaws to soften.

4. Note the contrast between tension and relaxation. . . . Allow the relaxation to spread and penetrate all over your face, your forehead and scalp, eyes, jaws, lips, tongue, and neck muscles.

5. Continue to move the relaxation down your body by tightening and then softening each muscle group. Notice the contrast of tight and soft, and how your body feels as it releases the tightness.

Exercise Two

1. Put your hand on your forehead and apply pressure by pushing your head into your hand. Feel the tension in your neck. Continue this pressure as you roll your head to the right and notice the tension shift. . . . Now roll it to the left. Release the pressure against your hand and then press your chin toward your chest. Breathe. Let your head return to a comfortable position, and notice the relaxation. Let the relaxation develop, increase, deepen, and flow.

2. Shrug your shoulders up. Hold the tension. . . . Drop your shoulders and feel the relaxation in your neck and shoulders. . . . Shrug your shoulders again and move them around. Bring your shoulders up . . . and forward . . . and back. Tighten the muscles and feel the tension in your shoulders and in your upper back. Drop your shoulders once more, breathe, and relax.

3. Let the relaxation spread deep into the shoulders . . . and into your back muscles. . . . Relax your neck and throat and jaws and other facial areas as the peaceful relaxation takes over and grows deeper . . . deeper . . . even deeper.

Exercise Three

1. Focus your attention on your forehead. Breathe, softening the muscles in your forehead.

2. Breathe, softening your eyes and your eyelids.

3. Breathe, softening your cheeks.

4. Breathe, softening your jaws.

5. Breathe, softening your neck muscles.

6. Breathe, softening all the muscles between your neck and your shoulders.

7. Breathe, softening your shoulders.

8. Breathe, softening your upper arms.

9. Breathe, softening your elbows.

10. Breathe, softening your lower arms.

11. Breathe, softening your wrists.

12. Breathe, softening your hands.

13. Breathe, softening your fingers.

14. Breathe, softening your fingertips.

15. Breathe, softening your chest and rib cage.

16. Just slightly notice your breathing, letting your body breathe all by itself.

17. Breathe, softening your stomach and buttocks.

18. Breathe, softening your thighs.

19. Breathe, softening your knees.

20. Breathe, softening your calves.

21. Breathe, softening your ankles.

22. Breathe, softening your feet.

23. Breathe, softening your toes.

Throughout this exercise, you may notice that your arms and legs feel heavier, or they might feel lighter. You may also feel a pleasant tingling sensation in your arms or legs. Become familiar with the sensations in your body as it relaxes. Let these sensations become deeper and stronger.

Become aware of how your body feels as you breathe out. Notice how the pleasant, tingling sensations seem to be stronger when you exhale. Imagine that you are letting go of all the tension with each exhalation. Let go of any active thoughts as well.

Return your focus to each step of the relaxation, or focus on your breathing. If music is playing in the background, focus on the music.

Remember how it felt to relax. As you go about your usual activities throughout the day, try to reproduce this feeling with your breathing.

Autogenics Training

The benefits of autogenics are similar to those of other meditative and relaxation techniques. Muscle tension decreases, blood flows more easily to the extremities. People who have migraines, Raynaud's, and insomnia have shown documented improvements with this technique. Autogenics means "self-generated," and you'll find it a powerful tool.

You will use the sensations of heaviness and warmth to achieve relaxation. Get into a relaxed position in a quiet location. Memorize and repeat the statements in this exercise. Or, have someone with a soothing voice read these directions into a tape recorder. This way, you can close your eyes, get comfortable, and concentrate on the directions.

Do not try to force yourself to feel heavy or warm, but remain unconcerned about what you feel. The phrases will work whether you feel anything or not. There is no right way to feel.

1. Start by going through all the phrases (this should take a few minutes):
   · My right arm is heavy . . . my left arm is heavy.
   · Both my arms are heavy.
   · My right leg is heavy . . . my left leg is heavy.
   · Both my legs are heavy.
   · My arms and legs are heavy.
   · My right arm is warm . . . my left arm is warm.
   · Both my arms are warm.
   · My right leg is warm . . . my left leg is warm.
   · Both my legs are warm.
   · My arms and legs are warm.
   · My arms and legs are heavy and warm.

2. Repeat the entire sequence to deepen your relaxation. You might repeat it a number of times to give your mind something to focus on.

3. To end the session, take a deep breath, stretch, and open your eyes.

Eventually, just saying the first phrase, "My right arm is heavy," followed by "My arms and legs are heavy and warm," will be enough to cue your body to enter a passive, relaxed state.

If you feel uncomfortable during this process, stop. Don't try this exercise again until meeting with your healthcare provider.

Breathing Exercises

Choose your favorite general breathing technique from the following list. Repeat this exercise slowly for several minutes, then move on to the deep natural breathing exercise on page 15. Or, for a more focused breathing technique, try mindful breathing, described on page 16.

General Breathing Techniques

4/4 Breathing

1. Count to 4 while breathing in,

2. Count to 4 while holding your breath,

3. Count to 4 while breathing out,

4. Count to 4 while holding your breath.

6/3 Breathing

1. Count to 6 while breathing in,

2. Count to 3 while holding your breath,

3. Count to 6 while breathing out,

4. Count to 3 while holding your breath.

8/4 Breathing

1. Count to 8 while breathing in,

2. Count to 4 while holding your breath,

3. Count to 8 while breathing out,

4. Count to 4 while holding your breath.

Sequential Breathing

1. Count to 2 while breathing in,

2. Count to 2 while breathing out,

3. Count to 3 while breathing in,

4. Count to 3 while breathing out,

5. Count to 4 while breathing in,

6. Count to 4 while breathing out.

Hollow Body Breathing

1. Imagine that your body is hollow.

2. With each in-breath, slowly fill the hollow body with relaxation.

3. Breathe out to empty the hollow body.

Color Breathing

1. Picture your breath as a soft, relaxing color.

2. Breathe this color into all parts of your body.

Body Breathing

Breathe the relaxation:

1. Up one side of your body and down the other.

2. Up the front of your body and down the back.

3. Up through the soles of your feet to your head.

4. Throughout the inside of your body.

5. Down from the top of your head, over your skin, and back into your feet.

Deep Natural Breathing

Deep natural breathing can be done without calling any attention to yourself. You can use this technique whenever you feel stressed. It allows you the opportunity to relax and gather your thoughts. Practice this technique for 3 to 4 minutes.

1. Sit comfortably with feet uncrossed.

2. Place one hand on your chest and the other on your abdomen.

3. Inhale deeply through your nose, allowing your abdomen to expand and push your lower hand outward.

4. When the abdomen is extended, allow your chest to expand and push the upper hand outward.

5. Hold the air in for a couple of seconds.

6. As you begin to exhale slowly, concentrate on creating a whooshing sound through pursed lips.

7. Repeat several times in a slow, deliberate manner.

Mindful Breathing

Mindfulness is the practice of being totally present to the moment. Mindful breathing allows you to focus on the breath—the way the air moves in and out of your nose and mouth, the way your chest rises and falls—and continually bring yourself back to the breath when your thoughts begin to wander. Mindful breathing for 10 to 30 minutes every day can help you let go of thoughts and other irritations in your life. Start with 5 minutes and increase until you are comfortable with 15 to 20 minutes, or longer.

1. Sit or lie in a comfortable, well-supported position.

2. Focus on your breathing. Let go of all thoughts, feelings, body sensations, and sounds. Notice your in-breath and out-breath. Do not try to breathe in any particular way. Let your body breathe as it needs to breathe.

3. Continue to focus on your breath while you let go of all other awareness. When your thoughts are too demanding, say a phrase with each in-breath and out-breath. For example, on the in-breath say "I am," and on the out-breath say "relaxed." Or, you might say a prayer or words that will reinforce relaxation, like "peace" on the in-breath and "love" on the out-breath.

Music Relaxation

Music can be used to restore, maintain, and improve mental and physical health. Because it interacts with specific parts of the brain, it can elicit emotion, alter mood, and create physiological changes (affecting heart rate, respiration, and skin temperature, for example). To enhance relaxation, you can play music while doing any of the exercises in this book. Choosing music to manage pain and stress is quite simple. Try the following:

· Choose music you enjoy.
· Play music that has a slow, gentle, soothing sound. A rhythm that is slower than your heartbeat will help you relax, while one that is faster than your heartbeat will energize you.
· Allow your mind to explore the sounds and mood of the music.

- Listen to music at home or alone.
- Pretend to conduct the music.
- Use relaxing music as part of your breathing or relaxation exercises.
- Attend a concert.
- Sing, hum, or learn to play an instrument. Amuse yourself, have a little fun, make life interesting.
- Write a song about yourself.
- Make up a dance to music, or simply wiggle your fingers or tap your toes.

Visual Imagery

These techniques use thoughts, pictures, and the imagination to develop images of safety and healing. Throughout these exercises, use your five senses to imagine yourself seeing (colors, objects, and arrangements), hearing (sounds or silence), smelling (odors or fragrances), touching (objects and physical sensations), and tasting (flavors).

Before you perform any of the exercises in this section, it's important to find a quiet space where you won't be disturbed. Go to a favorite place where you can feel comfortable and safe. Then:

- imagine a pleasant light that can speed up healing. Imagine this light entering your body. Or,
- imagine a safe, peaceful place. Allow yourself to rest in this special place. If any unpleasant thoughts come up that are connected to this place, simply imagine a new and more comforting scene. Or,
- remember a favorite place you've visited. Imagine each detail vividly. Let yourself feel comfortable and relaxed in this safe place.

Once you are fully relaxed in your safe space, try any of the following exercises. Choose a favorite exercise and practice it every day, whether or not you are experiencing a pain flare.

Sandbag Imagery

This technique may be used to relieve pain in one area at a time. If your pain occurs in several areas of your body, decide which area of discomfort you want to relieve first.

1. Get into a well-supported, comfortable position. You may want to lie down or use a reclining chair.

2. Close your eyes, unless you feel better with them open. Most people can concentrate better with their eyes closed.

3. A brief relaxation technique at the beginning may be helpful, especially if you feel tense or find it hard to concentrate. Try one of the general relaxation exercises starting on page 6.

4. Breathe in slowly and deeply. Breathe out slowly. Continue to breathe slowly and evenly in whatever way is comfortable. This may be all that is needed to help you feel reasonably calm and comfortable.

5. Imagine that your body is an empty sack or bag.

6. Imagine slowly filling the bag with sand. Feel your body get heavier and heavier as this happens. You may begin anywhere. For example, you might imagine filling your body from your toes up to your head. You may want to think of each area of your body as it fills with sand and gets heavier.

7. Continue filling the sandbag (your body) until it is completely full of sand.

8. When the sandbag is completely full, focus on the location of your pain. If another person is available to help you, signal for him or her to

place one hand on top of the painful area and the other hand underneath. If this is impossible or uncomfortable, ask your assistant to place his or her hands near the pain instead. Either technique will help you focus on your pain. (Be sure to work out the instructions with your assistant in advance.)

9. Imagine making a small slit in the sandbag, at or near the area of pain.

10. Imagine the sand slowly trickling out.

11. Begin to imagine the pain trickling out slowly with the sand.

12. Continue visualizing the sand and pain slowly trickling out until the sandbag is completely empty, flat, depleted, and weightless.

13. Repeat these steps for each area of pain.

You may wish to develop an image of your pain, visualizing its color, size, weight, temperature, sound, texture (for example, sharp or jagged around the edges), or smell. You may then imagine these sensory images changing or leaving the body as the sandbag empties.

Red Ball of Pain Imagery

This exercise will take 10 to 20 minutes.

1. Scan your body and imagine gathering any pains, aches, or other symptoms into a ball.

2. Begin to change the size of the ball. Allow it to get bigger. How big can you make it? Now make it smaller. How small can you make it? Is it possible to make it the size of a grain of sand?

3. Next, allow the ball to move slowly out of your body, then farther away each time you exhale. Notice the pain moving away with each out-breath.

4. Change the size of the ball several times in both directions. This not only serves as a distraction from the pain, but helps you to manipulate the pain experience rather than feel trapped or overwhelmed by it. It provides a tremendous sense of control as well as pain relief.

Transforming Pain Imagery

As you begin this exercise, have three pieces of paper handy. Identify the area of pain you would like to work on, then draw three pictures of your pain.

Drawing 1: The pain or discomfort at its very worst.

Drawing 2: The pain or discomfort at its best, though still present.

Drawing 3: Your body in complete comfort when all your pain is gone.

Sit in a comfortable chair. During your imagery, you will move through all three drawings, imagining your pain at its worst, then imagining the pain steadily decreasing until there is no pain at all.

1. When you are ready to begin, get into a comfortable position and allow yourself to fully relax. When you feel ready, allow the image of your first drawing to come to mind. Do not experience the pain, but notice all that you can about the drawing.

2. When you are ready, move to your second drawing, noticing all that you can about it. What feels different from the first drawing?

3. Now, let go of the second drawing and notice the third. Pay close attention to how your body feels. What is different? Focus on this pain-free state. Take that feeling and play with it a little . . . make it brighter and clearer.

4.   Keeping this comfort and pleasure, know that you can recall this third image whenever you need to. What can you take from this experience to bring you back to the positive feelings of this third picture?

5.   When you are ready, allow yourself to return to the room you're in, bringing with you that complete feeling of comfort and absence of pain. Feel the chair you are sitting in, hear the noises around you, and, when you are ready, open your eyes and stretch. Feel the comfort you have brought from your third picture as you move through your day.

Glove Anesthesia

This pain control technique is most effective when pain is localized, as with headaches, muscle tightness, tension, or cramping. Determine which hand can be easily placed over the painful area. You will learn to numb your hand and transfer this numbness to the area that hurts.

1.   Sit as comfortably as you can in a chair, making sure your back is well supported. Now, begin to relax. Take a few deep, relaxing breaths. Breathe in through your nose . . . and out through your

mouth . . . letting each breath relax you a little bit more. Let your eyelids gently close, if they have not done so already. When they do, you can relax a little more deeply, letting your body enjoy whatever level of relaxation you are already experiencing.

2. Now imagine a bucket filled with clear, clean, ice-cold water sitting next to the hand you will be numbing. This healing water is kept cold with lots of ice cubes, and the water is in a shiny new metal bucket. Notice the details of this bucket; see the tiny water drops condensing on the outside of the container, the color of the bucket, the size.

3. You may wish to add something to the imaginary water, like a color, a secret ingredient, or an anesthetic solution such as novocaine. Prepare the water so it is just the right potency. You may feel your hand begin to tingle in eager anticipation.

4. When you are ready, lift up your hand and place it in your imaginary bucket. You might plunge the whole hand right into the solution, or you might gradually dip your fingertips, fingers, and palm until the entire hand is submerged. Imagine the tingling, cold numbness

immediately come into your hand. Feel it traveling from your fingertips to your wrist, like a glove of anesthesia. Experience the sensation of pins and needles, like when your hand goes to sleep.

5.   Go ahead and swirl your hand around in the water. Spread your fingers and hear the ice cubes clinking around.

6.   Notice any other unique sensations in your hand while the numbness and anesthesia become a part of your body. As you are getting ready to transfer this numbness, know that the rest of your body can remain warm and relaxed.

7.   Lift your numbed hand out of the ice-cold water and move it to the area of discomfort. Feel the numbness from your hand begin to transfer, as if the area of discomfort were a sponge soaking up the cold, numbing relief. . . . That's right, let all the numbness drain out of your hand and into the tissues where it is needed. . . . Feel that cold, tingling, numb sensation completely replace any last bit of discomfort. Feel the relief. Enjoy the comfort.

8. Return your hand to your healing solution and repeat this transfer technique. The numbing of your hand will occur twice as fast, and the power to numb and relieve the area of discomfort will be twice as potent.

9. When this second transfer is complete, let your hand rest comfortably in your lap, resuming normal sensation and temperature. Put away your imaginary bucket of ice water so you can use it again whenever you wish to recreate this relief. Be proud of what your mind and body have accomplished, and notice how long this comfort lasts.

10. When you are ready, take a deep, energizing breath, then open your eyes, feeling relaxed and comfortable.

Spirituality and Reflection

Thoughts and Stress

It is important to understand that negative thoughts activate a stress response in the body. Thoughts like "Tomorrow is going to be a terrible day," "Nobody loves me," "I should have done this," or "I can't deal with this pain" convey to your nervous system that a painful or intolerable situation is occurring or is about to occur. Your nervous system reacts as if your very survival is threatened, and it activates the stress response.

Using relaxation techniques, you can reverse the body's reaction to perceived danger and stop the spiral of negativity. You can learn to let go of stressful thoughts, become a neutral observer of the people and events in your life, and stay in the present moment. There is no need to worry or fantasize about misfortunes that probably will never happen. When a problem threatens to overwhelm you, you can learn to focus on one small piece at a time, dealing with no more than you can realistically handle today.

Thinking about painful memories also will activate the stress response. When you remember painful feelings, you reexperience them, and your body reacts. Notice and honor these feelings when they come up. Do one of the breathing exercises beginning on page 12, and make a conscious choice to let the painful feelings go, reframing the uncomfortable memories into pleasant ones. This will reduce your stress and allow you to become more relaxed. Try it!

Enhancing Spirituality

Spiritual health is important to recovery and overall well-being. It can give you a feeling of peace inside. In fact, prayer or meditation can be especially helpful to those who struggle with why the pain has happened to them. When faced with an accident or trauma, however, many people experience a spiritual crisis—they question their faith and begin to search for a deeper meaning and purpose in life. Through their spirituality, chronic pain sufferers can make sense of or give meaning to their suffering. They can focus on how the experience has helped them to grow.

Relying on the strength of your spiritual beliefs may not change your circumstances, but it can alter the way you perceive your situation and how you will respond. Knowing that a greater force is at work in your life may help to eliminate stressful feelings of being all alone with your pain. When you acknowledge that you are not the center of the universe, and that your emotional pain is, in part, spiritual, you begin to turn your eyes toward the spiritual, both within and without. You can then start to understand your place in the universal scheme, feeling a connection to all things and to an entity greater than yourself. This is the beginning of spiritual wellness, which is so vital to mind/body recovery.

You can make the following choices:

1. Begin to make peace with your past.

2. Forgive yourself for the mistakes you have made.

3. Make a commitment to yourself to go forward with your life despite the pain.

4. Work to enhance your spiritual awareness. For example, chanting, meditation, repetitious prayer, silent conversation, or focusing on a sacred object will all help you develop your spiritual side.

You might compare spirituality to the electricity that powers your home. You can fill your rooms with many new appliances, but until you plug them in, they do not function. Without a connection to the spirit, we do not fully function, either. We find ourselves dissatisfied and restless. The energy of spirituality is represented in the fullness of life. This collective energy is available to everyone—but we must choose to connect ourselves to the source.

People who suffer chronic pain experience an accumulation of all the pain that a particular injury has given. It is not only the pain of the moment, but also the pain of the past and of the future. Suffering changes, however, when you challenge the belief that your hurt will persist beyond the limits of patience or endurance. Suffering will also change when you discover (or rediscover) the energy of spirituality.

When you learn to work with the pain in the present moment, you can detach it from both the past and the future. Detachment reduces it to something less overwhelming. The pain will not take over.

Humor Medicine

We have all heard the old adage, "Laughter is the best medicine." Research is proving this to be true in a number of ways.

Our bodies were created to take care of themselves. When we slow down enough to listen to our bodies and to practice what makes us feel good, we are healthier and happier.

One of the body's healing mechanisms is laughter. Laughter releases chemicals into the body that boost the immune system, increase blood flow, and lower blood pressure. Laughter also releases "bad" emotions that cause harmful effects on the body. Laughter affects mood; it can brighten a bad day or lighten a stressful situation. It also creates a diversion from pain. While laughter cannot cure chronic illness, it is an effective tool in its treatment. Try to integrate regular laughter into your daily routine:

- Collect videos that are tried-and-true laugh stimulators, such as Lucille Ball episodes, Three Stooges movies, or Gallagher performances. Individual preferences will vary, of course.
- Collect jokes. Subscribe to a daily online joke service, read cartoons in the daily paper, and buy

joke books. Keep recipe cards or a notebook
with funny lines that always get you laughing.
· Practice laughing in front of the mirror.
· Make daily laughing a habit. Try to aim for at least
fifteen good belly laughs a day.

Set Aside Time to Focus on What Is

The world is not defined by pain, nor is it defined by
suffering. Staying mindful and enjoying the details of
the moment is healing.

Watch sunlight shining through the window. Notice
how the light falls on the dust particles in the air, how
the dust swirls with the air currents, how the particles
are framed by the windowpane.

Look into a fish tank and watch how effortlessly the
fins move, allowing the fish to glide in one direction,
then another. Watch how the fish explore every inch of
the tank. Place your mind with the fish and go with
each movement.

Observe your favorite plant. Notice how the leaves
move with the wind or the air currents. The color isn't
just one shade of green, but many. Inspect the top of a
leaf, then, very slowly and gently, turn the leaf to look
underneath. Notice how the leaf comes in contact with

your fingers. When you release it, watch how it falls from your fingers and hangs alone. The stem of the plant has a different texture than the leaves. Imagine the roots under the soil, bringing moisture and food to the rest of the plant.

These quiet, gentle explorations not only allow time for inner reflection, but also enhance our connection to the world around us.

Share Your Stress

Flares in your pain can often bring back all the negative feelings you've experienced through past trauma, illness, injury, treatment, or relationships.

It helps to talk to someone about your concerns and worries. Choose a person who will listen without judgment. Talking with a friend, family member, teacher, or counselor can help you see your problem in a different light. Knowing when to ask for help may allow you to avoid more serious problems later.

Journaling

A journal is a good place to voice dreams, disappointments, plans, and concerns. Many people think they are too busy to write in a journal, or they are afraid to write down their thoughts and feeling. Journaling, however, takes little time, and it is an effective weapon against pain and stress. It can help you:

· Release frustrations that you may not feel comfortable sharing with others.
· Identify recurrent feelings and thoughts.
· Get to know yourself better.
· Realize that there are other aspects to your life besides your pain and its effects.

Keeping a journal can be as simple or as difficult as you make it. There is no right or wrong way to journal. Here are some simple tips to get you started:

· Keep a notebook just for journaling.
· Find a quiet and comfortable place where you can write.
· Schedule a time for writing each day (every morning or evening, for example).
· Don't try to write the Great American Novel. It's fine to write just a sentence or two about how you are feeling and where your thoughts are that day. You don't need to come to any conclusions or make any profound discoveries. Just write what you are feeling and thinking.

To overcome your writer's block, try answering three questions each day: What did you experience today that you really enjoyed? What did you experience that you didn't enjoy? What did you experience that was new to you, and how did it feel? Remember, the simple act of writing down a thought, emotion, or problem can often help you feel better and develop new plans for coping.

Distraction

Distractions can help you function despite your pain. The art of distraction doesn't work in the same manner every time. Sometimes you need a gentle distraction, other times you need something a little more jarring.

Try the following strategies:
- Change activities. When your current activity becomes uncomfortable, do something else for a while. For example, if you are doing something sedentary, like writing, change gears and distract yourself with an active task, like watering plants.
- Listen to music. "Music hath charms to soothe the savage breast, to soften rocks, or bend a knotted

oak." It can also help you cope with pain. Refer to "Music Relaxation" on page 17.

· Draw something meaningful, or draw the pain. Refer to "Transforming Pain Imagery" on page 22.

Put Your Body Back to Work

Exercise

When you have chronic pain, the primary goal of exercise is to improve your ability to do normal daily activities. By adding physical activity to your routine, you get a sense that you can carry out an exercise program. This helps to remove the fear associated with movement. Other benefits of exercise include:

- a greater sense of relaxation,
- a more positive outlook,
- improved circulation and muscle endurance,
- improved movement without increased pain,
- reduction in the frequency and intensity of pain, and
- control over pain.

Furthermore, when you are nervous, angry, or upset, you can release these feelings through physical activity. Remember, your mind and your body work together.

You should include three forms of exercise in your weekly exercise routine: aerobic conditioning, strengthening, and stretching. First, though, you should seek approval from your primary care provider before starting an exercise program. Your healthcare provider can help you set reasonable exercise goals so that you will eventually meet your functional goals. If exercise causes serious discomfort or a worsening of symptoms, check with your doctor, nurse practitioner, or physical therapist. You may need to reevaluate your exercise plan and start another type of exercise.

Aerobic Exercises

Aerobic activity not only increases your breathing and heart rate, it releases chemicals in the body that naturally reduce pain. Examples of aerobic exercise include running, walking, playing tennis, and working in your garden.

Warm up with your aerobic exercise for 2 to 3 minutes, remain active for 15 to 20 minutes, and cool down by reducing your pace for 3 to 5 minutes. Some individuals will need to start with shorter periods of activity and gradually increase the duration over time. Remember to pace yourself.

Strengthening Exercises

By developing stronger muscles, you will increase your endurance, reduce your chances of reinjury, and improve the way you sit, stand, and move.

To strengthen your muscles, you will need light weights to provide resistance to your movement. You can create weights out of everyday household items, such as soup cans, detergent bottles (1/2-filled with water or sand), or a book bag filled with various weighted objects.

Warm up with aerobic activity for 3 to 5 minutes prior to strength training. For specific strengthening exercises, see your physical therapist.

Stretching Exercises

A key component of pain management, stretching stimulates your body's relaxation response. It is best to follow the stretching recommendations of your physical therapist. Stretching helps with:

- range of motion,
- joint flexibility (moving the joint fluid and surrounding joint structures),

- circulation of blood flow and other fluid in muscle tissue,
- muscle relaxation,
- balance and posture, and
- lifting and moving without increased pain.

Gentle stretches should be held for a minimum of 30 seconds and repeated 2 to 3 times. Stretches should be done daily—on comfortable days as well as painful days. Limit the force of your stretches when increased pain or swelling is present. Remember:

- Talk to your primary care provider before starting an exercise program.
- You may be sore after the first few times you exercise. This is normal and will get better with time.
- Be gentle with yourself.
- Pace yourself.
- Don't be competitive. No one is keeping score.
- Don't compare yourself to anyone else.

Every body has its limits. Know yours.

Pacing

Pacing is a technique you can use to prevent unnecessary pain flare-ups. Essentially, pacing means interrupting your work or activity for short, frequent breaks. For example, it is much better to take a 10-minute break each hour than to take a 30-minute break every 2 to 3 hours. Taking a break allows you to change your position and relieve stress on your muscles and joints, thereby breaking the cycle of stress, muscle tension, and pain.

You can minimize the possibility of unnecessary pain flares by following these simple guidelines:

- Plan scheduled breaks and stick to the schedule.
- Alternate easy and difficult tasks throughout the day or week.
- If you absolutely cannot take a break, try to interrupt the activity and change your body position as frequently as possible. For example, if you have been sitting at a computer, stand up and stretch for a few minutes. If you have been standing, sit and stretch every chance you get.
- Change positions before you feel fatigued or sore.
- Practice deep breathing for relaxation.
- Stop to stretch frequently, approximately every 10 to 15 minutes.
- Take your time to avoid feeling rushed and anxious.

Let go of the pressure to do everything at once. To integrate pacing skills into your life, try the following:

Gather three blank pieces of paper. On one piece, write a list of things you absolutely have to do. On another, write a list of things you should do. On the third piece, write a list of things you love to do. Each day, do two things from each list, no more. Cross them off when you are finished. If you can't do two things from each list, try again tomorrow. The goal is to pace yourself.

Energy Conservation

Normal, everyday activities can be difficult for those who have chronic pain. By conserving your energy throughout the day, you will reduce the frequency and intensity of pain flares. When combined with the pacing technique, energy conservation can become an essential part of your pain management plan. Remember the following:

- Eliminate unnecessary tasks.
- Avoid unnecessary bending, reaching, or walking.
- When possible, avoid lifting objects by sliding them along a counter or using a cart.
- Pack grocery bags so they aren't too heavy, and place them in a rolling cart when possible.
- Do not overload purses and briefcases.
- Avoid using shoulder bags, as these may throw off your balance and cause more muscular pain.

Body Mechanics

The manner in which you maintain your posture, or body position, at rest or during activity is called body mechanics. Without proper body mechanics, injury or pain flare are more likely to occur.

Learning to remain aware of your body and to move properly can be labor intensive. It will take time and practice to incorporate the proper techniques into your daily life.

There are three principles of body mechanics:

1. Distribute the force of any activity throughout your whole body. In other words, be aware of any tense muscles in your body, then work to relax those muscles using the techniques discussed in this book. Keep in mind that if one area of the body holds more tension than another, energy is absorbed above and below that area, increasing the chance of injury. For example, if you move while your hip muscles are tense, your knees and lower back will be at risk.

2. Pay attention to your posture. Because your body absorbs the force of every movement you make, poor posture increases your chance of pain and injury. You can reduce this risk by maintaining

proper body alignment. In other words, practice keeping your body in a neutral position.

The neutral position of the spine is achieved when the nose is in line with the belly button, and the ear, shoulder, and hip are on a vertical line when viewed from the side.

The neutral position of the head and neck controls the curve of the neck. The ears are over the shoulders, the eyes are level, and the chin is tucked in slightly.

The neutral position of the shoulders controls the curve in the mid-back. The shoulders are directly over the hips, and the rib cage is elevated away from the abdomen, allowing you to breathe from the diaphragm.

The neutral position of the pelvis controls the curve in the low back. If too little curve is present, the top of the pelvis can be tilted forward, thereby slightly increasing the curve in the back. If too much of a curve exists, rolling the top of the pelvis back and tightening the abdominal muscles will correct this.

Try to remain aware of your body. If you continually practice these positions, they will eventually become automatic. If you're not sure about a position, check with a healthcare professional.

3. Break difficult activities into separate movements. The following exercise, called the Waiter's Bow, demonstrates this concept.
    - Pause to relax your hips, knees, and ankles. (Always do this before you begin to bend or squat.)
    - Check your trunk alignment.
    - Place your hands on a countertop.
    - Bend forward at the hips.
    - Your back should remain straight. Do not arch your back.
    - Allow your hips to sway back slightly.
    - Return to an upright position.

What to Do When
Your Pain Flares

Most of the techniques described in this book will help you decrease pain levels over time, and sometimes prevent pain altogether. Pain cannot always be prevented, however. When it does occur, it's important to know how to control it. Try the following methods to see what works best for you.

Cultivating Endorphins

When the body experiences short-term pain, the brain releases natural chemicals called endorphins. The word *endorphin* comes from *endo* (meaning "produced within") and *orphine* (having a chemical structure similar to morphine). Endorphins have a wide variety of beneficial effects on the body, such as relieving pain, elevating mood, and boosting the immune system. Chronic stress, alcohol and drug abuse, and frequent narcotic use will all suppress endorphins.

When the body senses pain, glands in the body release endorphins into the bloodstream. The endorphins are then picked up by receptor sites in the brain, along the spinal column, and in other areas of the body. Once the endorphins connect with their pain-producing targets in the body, the sensation of pain is modified and the experience of pain is reduced.

While pain may cause your body to naturally release endorphins, it is possible to "cultivate endorphins" before, during, or after a pain flare. This will increase the number of endorphins in your body and further reduce your pain. There are a number of ways to cultivate endorphins:

- Spend time in nature (especially in sunshine).
- Surround yourself with supportive friends and family members.
- Eat well-balanced meals.
- Write, draw, play music, or use other creative outlets to express yourself.
- Laugh. In his wonderful book, *Anatomy of an Illness*, Norman Cousins demonstrates that laughter is an excellent way to release endorphins.

· Exercise. When joggers experience a "runner's high," they are feeling the effects of endorphins. Endorphins can also be released through yoga, tai chi, chi gong, and other physical activities.

Cold and Hot Packs

Cold

Cold is best for red, hot, or swollen joints and muscles. It is used to reduce inflammation and swelling, relax tense muscles, and numb the painful area. Generally, cold is recommended for the first 24 to 48 hours after an injury.

Good sources of cold include:
- · an ice pack wrapped in a damp towel,
- · a bag of frozen peas, or
- · a Zip-Loc bag filled with ice cubes and then wrapped in a damp towel.

Apply cold to the affected area for 10 to 15 minutes, two to three times a day. If you are using ice or a cold pack from the freezer, place a towel between the cold pack and your skin. If you experience skin irritation or an increase in symptoms, discontinue the cold pack and consult your doctor.

Heat

Heat helps relieve joint stiffness, muscle spasms, and pain. It relaxes tense muscles and increases blood flow. Moist heat is best. Generally, heat is recommended 48 to 72 hours after an injury has occurred, but it can also provide great comfort during a pain flare.

Good sources of heat include:

- a moist heating pad,
- a warm shower or bath, or
- a moist towel heated in a microwave.

Apply heat to the affected area for 15 to 20 minutes, two to three times a day. Remember to place a cloth between the hot pack and your skin. To prevent burns, heat should not be applied over an area of the body that has lost sensation (from diabetes or a stroke, for example). If you experience a burn or an increase in symptoms, discontinue use and consult your doctor.

TENS Unit Application

TENS (Transcutaneous Electrical Nerve Stimulation) can help control chronic pain and acute surgical pain. A TENS Unit is a small device that sends an electrical signal through the skin to the nerves that carry the pain message to your brain. When successful, the TENS Unit will "switch off" the pain message by stimulating certain nerves to override pain-carrying nerves, or by stimulating the pain-carrying nerves to block the pain message.

Using the TENS Unit

1. Turn the TENS Unit off before attaching or removing electrode pads or wires.

2. Place the electrode pads on the skin around the painful area or along the most tender points.

3. Attach the electrode wires to the TENS Unit.

4. Adjust the dials to a comfortable level.

5. Note the time. Be sure not to leave the TENS Unit on for more than two hours at once.

6. Leave the TENS Unit off for at least one hour between sessions to avoid muscle spasms and skin irritation.

7. Use the TENS Unit at least one hour before bedtime, then turn it off for the night to prevent skin irritation.

Precautions:

- Ask your doctor or physical therapist how often you may use the TENS Unit.
- Do not let anyone else use your TENS Unit.
- Keep electrode pad sites clean and dry.
- Check for signs of skin irritation under the pads every twenty-four hours.
- Alternate electrode pad sites at least every three days.
- Remove the pads and electrode wires for showering, bathing, or swimming.
- When removing an electrode pad, peel the edges back in the direction of hair growth. Application sites should be checked periodically for signs of skin irritation.
- Clip—don't shave—body hair around the electrode pad sites.
- Do not place electrode pads over cut or irritated skin.
- Do not stretch electrode pads over the skin.
- Try to position electrode pads so that the load wires are perpendicular to the direction of body movement. Have your physical therapist demonstrate this for you.
- Check your TENS Unit frequently to make sure the wires are securely connected and are not bent.

If skin irritation occurs:
  · Consult your doctor, physical therapist, or nurse to be sure the irritation is not related to the length of time the TENS Unit is kept on.
  · When possible, alter placement slightly when changing electrodes.
  · Discontinue TENS if you develop a rash or sore, then contact your doctor, physical therapist, or nurse.

Ball Therapy

Ball therapy is a pain relief technique used while lying on the floor or sitting in a chair. It requires one or more balls from 1 to 6 inches in diameter. Tennis balls or racquetballs work well.

Place a ball under or against any of the following painful areas: the head or neck; along either side of the spine in the upper back; under the pelvis on either side of the sacrum; under one or both knees; under the sole of the foot; or under the forearm or hand. Do not place the ball on any muscle or joint where it causes so much pain that you cannot relax your weight onto the ball.

The balls can be used two different ways:
  · for direct pressure on sore or spasmodic muscles, causing a release of tension, or

· as a point of instability, allowing you to explore movement in a slow, relaxed way. This also facilitates the release of tension in the surrounding joints and muscles.

When moving on a ball, do so as slowly as you can in all possible directions. Pause often to relax completely in different positions. Do not move through pain unless it is a "hurts-so-good" type of sensation.

Contrast Baths

Contrast baths are convenient when pain is located in the extremities (in the hands or feet, for example). The sore or injured body part is alternately bathed in hot and cold water, which leads to improved circulation, distraction from the pain, and relaxation of the muscles.

You will need:

· two small pans or tubs, 10 to 15 inches across (or one pan and a bathtub),
· a candy or meat thermometer (must register between 50° and 115° F), and
· a towel.

Procedure:

1. Fill one of the tubs with hot water. Never use water that is hotter than 106° F.

2. Fill the other tub with cold water (approximately 65° F, about the same temperature as the water that comes from a cold faucet).

3. Soak the injured area in hot water, then cold, alternating according to the following schedule:

    Hot: 10 minutes
    > Cold: 1 minute

    Hot: 4 minutes
    > Cold: 1 minute

    Hot: 4 minutes
    > Cold: 1 minute

    Hot: 4 minutes

    Total Time: 25 minutes

4. After the final 4-minute soak in hot water, dry your body well.

5. Massage the injured area with massage oil or sesame oil (available in the natural foods section at the grocery store).

Acupressure

Acupressure is one of many techniques associated with traditional Chinese medicine. For thousands of years, this medical system has been used to successfully treat much of the world's population.

Acupressure uses fingertip pressure on key areas of the body, called acupoints. The body contains about one thousand acupoints, most relating to specific organs. Applying pressure to these acupoints can decrease pain, nausea, and physical symptoms while facilitating emotional release and relaxation.

This technique has been used to treat physical, emotional, and spiritual challenges. It is a safe, effective tool that can be used along with (or in some cases in place of) medications. You can receive acupressure treatment from another person, or you can administer self-acupressure. In either case, acupressure is relatively painless and very relaxing.

How Does Acupressure Work?

Traditional Chinese medicine believes that when a person is healthy, energy flows smoothly through his or her body. An interruption or blockage in the flow of energy results in physical symptoms like pain, fatigue, nausea, muscle tightness, or cramps. Emotions that are repressed or ignored can also cause an imbalance in the energy flow, leading to symptoms like irritability, depression, frustration, stress, and a sense of being overwhelmed or out of control. Consistent imbalance can eventually cause disease.

The purpose of acupressure is to release the blockage of energy, readjust the flow, and help restore balance. For people with chronic pain, acupressure can be used to induce relaxation, loosen tight muscles, and reduce or relieve pain.

Traditional Chinese medicine focuses on the whole person. The foods we eat, the beverages we drink, the air we breathe, physical or emotional trauma, and environmental factors (heat, dampness, dryness, cold, wind) all influence the proper flow of energy. Acupressure helps restore the flow of energy so the body can heal itself; however, it cannot "fix" the person. To achieve optimum health, we must be willing to look at how our lives are unfolding. Our attention must be focused on balancing all areas of our lives and nurturing the body, mind, and soul.

Using Acupressure Points

Acupoints can be stimulated with direct pressure or massage. Pressure can be applied with the thumb, fingernail, thumbnail, tip of the index finger, or palm of the hand. Massage can be done using tiny circles at the rate of about two to three circles per second. Enough pressure should be used to massage the tissues beneath the skin.

Pressure will vary according to individual tolerance and preference. You should begin very slowly and gently, especially if you are sick, weak, or tired. If you desire more pressure, a gradual increase is best. When it is time to release the point, do so slowly. Acupoints will be tender and should "hurt so good," but the pressure should not be so great as to cause pain.

Generally, you should hold a point for 1 to 2 minutes, but longer or shorter periods may be more helpful. Pay attention to what you feel as you hold the point. Sometimes you will feel the muscle or tissue begin to soften and relax beneath your finger. You may feel a temperature change on the skin or notice changes in breathing, like a heavy sigh. These are signs that the body is relaxing. When the point is ready to be released, you may feel a subtle pulsing sensation under your finger. Again, release the pressure gradually. Remember:

· Acupressure is not a substitute for medical care. It is meant to complement medical science by assisting the body's healing process.
· Do not apply pressure to open wounds, bruises, sprains, or swelling. Gentle pressure above or below these areas can effectively assist the flow of energy and encourage self-healing.
· Do not use self-acupressure if you are pregnant or thinking about becoming pregnant.

Indications for Self-Acupressure

Insomnia

The long-term use of sleeping pills isn't always beneficial for a person with chronic pain. Regular self-acupressure, however, may help restore disrupted sleep patterns. To locate the relevant acupoints, use the diagrams on the following pages. You will notice that the points are tender when you press on them.

K6, called Joyful Sleep, is located directly below the inside of the anklebone, in a slight indentation. In addition to relieving insomnia, pressing this point eases anxiety, high blood pressure, and ankle and heel pain. The effect is enhanced when K6 is pressed at the same time as B62, Calm Sleep, which is located in the first indentation directly below the outer anklebone.

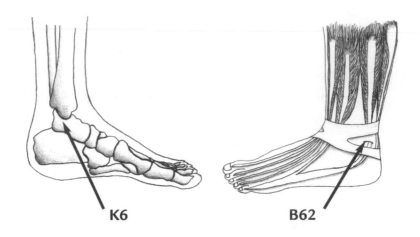

K6   **B62**

Traditional Chinese medicine holds that a troubled heart can prevent restful sleep. H7, or Spirit Gate, helps to calm the heart and relieve stress, anxiety, cold sweats, and insomnia resulting from overexcitement. When you bend your wrist, H7 is located below the palm of your hand, in the wrist crease under the bone on the little-finger side.

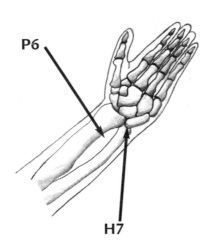

P6

H7

P6, Inner Gate, is located between the two tendons on the inner forearm, three finger widths down from the wrist crease. This point relieves anxiety, palpitations, indigestion, and an upset stomach. P6 is also known as the "master nausea point."

CV17, called Sea of Tranquillity, is located on the center of the breastbone. To find it, follow the bottom of the ribs to where they join in the center, then measure three finger widths until you reach a small indentation in the breastbone. CV17 relieves nervousness, chest congestion, and anxiety, all of which contribute to insomnia.

B38, called Vital Diaphragm, is located at heart level between the shoulder blades and the spine. This point calms intense emotions that may interfere with sleep.

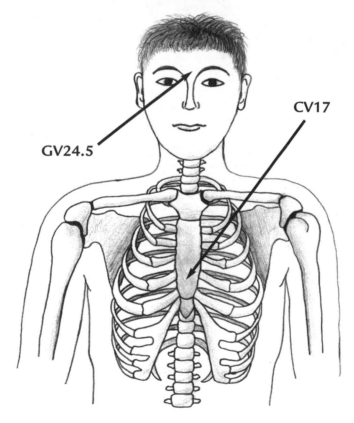

To put pressure on B38, lie on your back, placing a tennis ball or racquetball on each acupoint. Close your eyes and use the breathing and imagery techniques outlined in this book to induce relaxation.

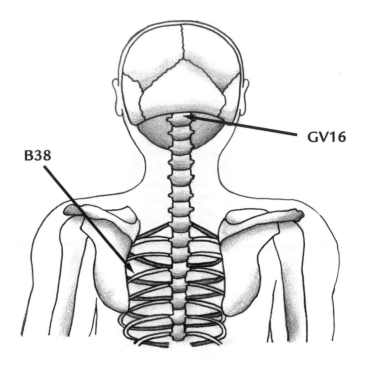

Pain

You may notice that when you are under stress, your pain becomes worse. Stress causes muscular tension and reduced blood flow, which leads to increased pain. Because acupressure relieves muscle tension and aids circulation, it can reduce and sometimes prevent pain.

Furthermore, acupressure releases endorphins, which not only help block the transmission of pain, but also elevate your mood.

A widely used point for general pain relief, Hoku, or LI4, can ease joint and muscular pain in the upper body. Find the sore spot between your thumb and forefinger where the bones join together. Hold the point firmly enough to produce tenderness for

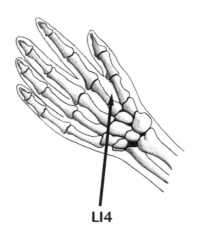

LI4

1 to 2 minutes. At the same time, flex the joint nearest the part of your body that's in pain. For instance, if your neck hurts, move your head up and down as you firmly press Hoku. After a minute or two, release the point and work on Hoku on your other hand. Again, move the joint that is closest to your pain while you firmly press LI4. After a few minutes, you may find that much of your pain is relieved. Stimulating this point can also relieve arthritis, constipation, headaches, toothaches, and shoulder pain. CAUTION: This point is forbidden for pregnant women until labor, because stimulation of this point can cause premature contractions in the uterus.

GV16, called Wind Mansion, is located at the back of the head in the large hollow at the base of the skull (see page 64). GV16 relieves headaches, stiff necks, and pain in the eyes, ears, nose, and throat. Combining this point with GV24.5 enhances the beneficial effects. Located directly between the eyebrows, GV24.5 is in the indentation where the bridge of the nose meets the forehead (see page 63). Hold each point and imagine breathing into your head, relaxing the chatter in your mind.

St36 is one of the most helpful points for lower body pain. Four finger widths below the kneecap, place your fingertips 1/2 inch outside the shinbone. If you are on the correct spot, you will feel a muscle flex as you move your foot up and down. Now, make a fist with both hands and place your knuckles on the St36 points on both legs. Briskly rub these points with your knuckles up and down along the outside of your shinbones. Breathe deeply as you rub these acupressure points for 1 minute. Drink one full glass of water upon completion of this exercise.

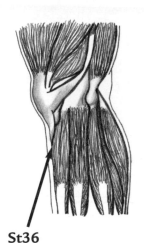

St36

Hand Massage

Hand massage can be an extremely effective tool to relieve pain and anxiety during a pain flare. By massaging certain parts of your hand, you can reduce pain in various parts of your body. There are no side effects to this technique; it is safe and can be used anywhere, even at work.

If the right side of your body hurts, massage your right hand. If the left side of your body hurts, massage the left hand.

Start with the lower part of the palm, near the wrist. Massage one hand with the other, using your thumb on the palm and supporting the back of the hand with your fingers. Gradually work your way around the entire palm. If your thumb becomes tired, use one or two fingers to massage while resting the back of your hand on a table or firm pillow.

Use a circular pressure, first clockwise, then counterclockwise. You need to push hard enough to feel the muscles and bones of your hand. If you notice that a particular part of your palm is tender, apply a firm, steady pressure on that point for a few seconds, then release. Try to remember where the tender spots are so you can massage them again later.

After you are done with the hand massage, drink one full glass of water.

Pain Management Plan

A pain management plan requires a strong commitment. You cannot always prevent a pain flare; however, by practicing the techniques described in this book, you can learn to manage your pain. Use this worksheet to develop your personal pain management plan. When you write down the plan in your own words, you will be more likely to follow through with it. It will take time and effort to reach your goals, and the journey may be frustrating and difficult, so keep your plan realistic. Post your plan near your desk, on the refrigerator, or in another visible area so you can be reminded of it often.

Consider the following questions:

How will you respond to your pain?

How long will it take to learn this response?

Visualize your response. What does it look like?

Afterward, ask yourself:

Was this response helpful?

Would I be able to respond this way to future pain flares?

Do I need to practice this response?

What would I do differently next time?

References

Congreve, William. *Mourning Bride*, act 1, scene 1. In *Familiar Quotations*, 10th edition, edited by John Bartlett. Boston: Little, Brown and Company, 1919.

Cousins, N. *Anatomy of an Illness*. New York: W.W. Norton and Company, 1979.

Davis, M., E. R. Eshelman, and M. McKay. *The Relaxation and Stress Reduction Workbook*. 3rd Edition. Oakland, Calif.: New Harbinger Publications, 1988.

Ezra, S. *Glove Anesthesia for Pain Control*. Foster City, Calif.: Beyond Ordinary Nursing, 1999.

Ezra, S., and T. Reed. *Beyond Ordinary Nursing*. Foster City, Calif.: Beyond Ordinary Nursing, 1999.

Ezra, S., and T. Reed. *Transforming Pain*. Foster City, Calif.: Beyond Ordinary Nursing, 1999.

Gach, M. R. *Acupressure's Potent Points*. New York: Japan Publications, 1981.

McCaffery, M., and C. Pasero. *Pain Clinic Manual*. 2nd Edition. St. Louis: Mosby, 1999.

Editors

Barbara St. Marie, MA, ANP, GNP   Susan Arnold, BA, RN, CHTP

Contributors

Barbara Alexander, RN, BS

David Alter, PhD, LP, ABPP

Kathleen Avila, MA, LP

Miles Belgrade, MD

Al Clavel, MD

Debra Drew, RN, MS

Ted Ellquist, LPT

Barbara Frankel, MPT

Paula Jelinek, RN, BA

Daly King, RN

Rebecca Maddox, RN, C

Roberta Moore, RN, MA, HNC

Steven Murray, MA

Patrick O'Laughlin, PhD, LP

Georgia Panopoulos, PhD, LP

Brenda Severson, RN, BS

James Struve, MD

Teresa Taylor, BA

Bobbie Walker, MA, LP

David Wilkening, LPT, CFP

Acknowledgments

Rich Boortz-Marx, MD

Virginia Glen, PharmD

Marty Heller, RN

Mark Stuckey, MD

Suzanne Proudfoot, DO

Bonnie Warner

Janet Wirmel